All About
FOOT CARE &
DIABETIC ULCERS

by Kenneth Wright

in consultation with Dr. Rory Gatenby D.P.M., F.A.C.F.A.O.M.

Member of American Board of

Podiatric Orthopedics & Primary Podiatric Medicine

Fellow of American College of Foot & Ankle Orthopedics & Medicine

Other contributors include the following nurse educators:

A special thanks to the American Association of Podiatrists for access to their patient educational material and advice on this book. Other contributors include: Canadian Association of Wound Care (CAWC), the Canadian Diabetes Association and the several wound care nurses both E.T.s and WOCN members who advised on the this project.

ISBN # 978-1-896616-87-2

© 2011, 2017 Mediscript Communications Inc.

Foot care. Diabetes. Diabetic Foot ulcers. Foot ulcers. Feet. Self help. Foot care.

First edition. All rights reserved

Printed in Canada

www.mediscript.net

Book and Front Cover design by:
Brian Adamson, www.AdamsonGraphics.net

FC1002011

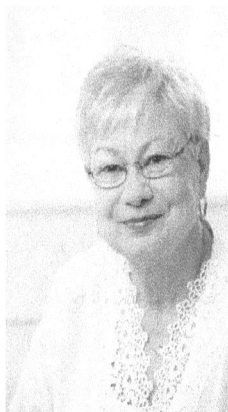

CONTENTS

INTRODUCTION

This book provides basic, non controversial and trusted information about foot care and the implications for foot health when someone has diabetes.

The objective of this book is to provide understanding about the role of diabetes in causing damage to the feet (e.g. foot ulcers), and subsequently being able to take actions and change lifestyle patterns in order to prevent this damage occurring.

Further, this book provides the essential ABC's of foot care which not only helps in the fight against damaging your feet if you have diabetes but provides general self help foot care tips for anybody wanting to ensure good overall foot health, thereby helping to prevent any future foot problems.

Health workers in nursing homes, home care agencies and hospitals will find in this book layman terminology and a down-to-earth perspective on the condition which will help for better understanding and assist in being able to communicate with clients and patients. As a health care professional you may in fact want to recommend that

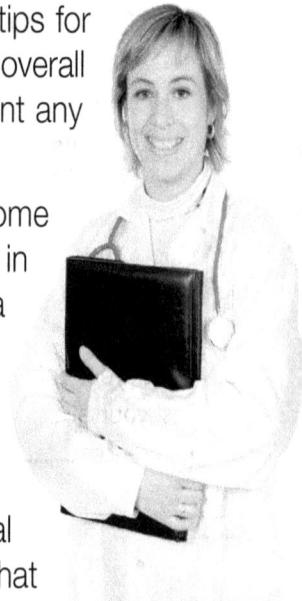

your patients or clients pick up a copy of the book.

All the information is reliable, and the information was obtained from authoritative bodies, adhering to best practice guidelines. Our group of nurse educators edited the book and the Internet version is HON (Health On the Net) certified, for your peace of mind.

SOMETHING TO THINK ABOUT...

Life's most persistent and urgent question is:

What are you doing for others?

Martin Luther King, Jr.

AN IMPORTANT MESSAGE
FROM THE PUBLISHER

Each person's treatment, advice, medical aids, physical therapy and other approaches to health care are unique and highly dependant upon the diagnosis and overall assessment by the medical team.

We emphasize therefore that the information within this book is not a substitute for the advice and treatment from a health care professional.

This book provides generic information about well established self care and self help tips for foot care with basic information on diabetes and how that condition contributes to foot ulcers.

With all this in mind, the publishers and authors disclaim any responsibility for any adverse effects resulting directly or indirectly from the suggestions contained within this book or from any misunderstanding of the content on the part of the reader.

HAVE YOU HEARD

Signs you are over the hill::

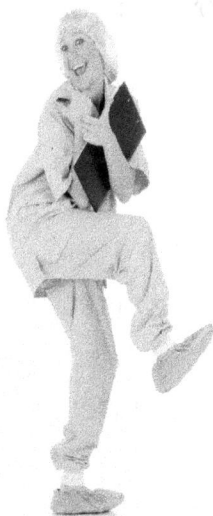

- You run out of breath walking down a flight of stairs.
- The speed limit seems excessive.
- Your back goes out more often than you do.
- The animals you had as a kid are extinct.
- At cafeterias, you complain the gelatin is too tough.

HOW MUCH DO YOU KNOW

1. Which of the following is not a foot care practice?

a. Daily wash and dry

b. Use a pleasant, perfumed lotion over any sore

c. Frequent toenail care

d. Regular foot inspection for danger signs

2. What is the best definition of diabetes?

a. A disease that is controlled mostly by injections of insulin

b. A person with diabetes has below average levels of glucose (sugar) in the blood

c. A disease usually inherited that affects the body's blood sugar (glucose) levels

d. A disease which has the characteristic of high blood sugar (glucose) levels

3. Which of the following diabetes complications is false?

a. Eye (retina) problems affecting vision

b. Cardiovascular (heart and circulation) problems

c. Foot ulcers

d. Hearing disability

4. For people at risk or who have a diabetic foot ulcer, foot inspection should take place:

a. Once a month

b. Once a week

c. Twice a day

d. At least twice a week

5. Which of the following is not a risk factor for developing a diabetic foot ulcer?

a. Smoking cigarettes

b. Overweight

c. Infrequent foot inspection

d. Too much exercise

6. Which of the following toenail care practices should not be done?

a. Cutting the toenail straight across

b. Use sharp scissors to cut toenails

c. Preferably cut toenails after a bath, when they are softer

d. Keep the lighting bright when cutting toenails

7. Which of the following activities can contribute to foot infection?

a. Walking barefoot

b. Regular foot inspection

c. Practicing good hygienic foot care practices

d. Bathing the foot in tepid instead of very hot water

ANSWERS

1. b. Using a scented lotion can cause irritation or an allergic reaction.

2. d. High blood sugar is the basic harmful characteristic of diabetes.

3. d. Hearing loss has never been associated with diabetes but the other 3 can be serious complications.

4. d. Twice a week on average is about right.

5. d. Too much exercise is usually not a risk factor unless it damages the feet.

6. b. Instead of sharp scissors, the use of nail clippers is recommended to avoid the risk of being cut.

7. a. Walking barefoot can cause unnecessary damage to the foot.

WHAT IS A FOOT ULCER

The most problematical diabetes complication as far as quality of life is concerned is the development of a foot ulcer. Apart from treatment issues and mobility problems there is always the risk of hospitalization and amputation of the foot or leg.

The following body components are associated with a foot ulcer:

NERVES: enable you to feel sensations like heat, cold, pressure, pain and irritations.

BLOOD VESSELS: transport oxygen and vital nutrients to nourish your feet and help them heal from injuries or sores.

BONES: give your foot shape and effectively distribute the pressure from your weight.

JOINTS: the mobile connections between your bones enabling your foot to move as well as absorb pressure.

SKIN: together with fat tissue it envelopes your foot, absorbing pressure and protecting your foot from infection.

When you have diabetes, the daily wear and tear on your feet can be more damaging than for a person without diabetes. The greatest damage is done to areas of your feet that take the most pressure.

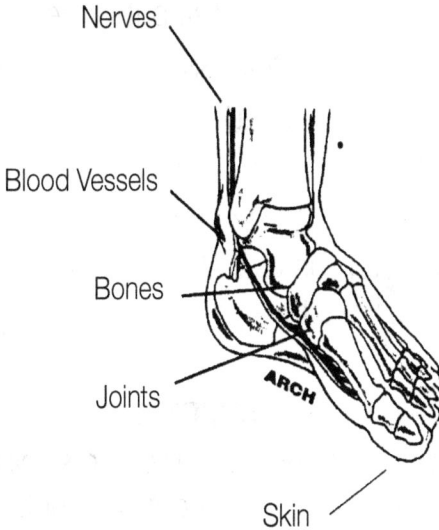

Here's a simple outline of what can go wrong:

NERVE DAMAGE: Diabetes causes your nerve cells to become damaged and non functional. This can make your feet feel numb – insensitive to heat, cold or pain. Consequently, you can injure your foot without knowing it.

CLOGGED-UP BLOOD VESSELS: The blood capillaries can become clogged-up and inefficient, meaning not enough blood is getting to the skin area. If the foot becomes damaged there may not be enough blood to provide the healing nutrients and chemicals necessary for quick healing.

WEAKENED BONES: These may slowly shift, making a foot somewhat deformed and thereby changing the way your foot distributes pressure.

WEAKENED JOINTS: The ability to absorb pressure is reduced, the arch may fall and skin may now start to break down.

SKIN BREAKDOWN: Pressure – something as innocuous as a stone in your shoe – can lead to sores developing and, if bacteria are present, infections will occur.

FOOT ULCER DEVELOPMENT: Skin breakdown can appear simply as warm or red spots, blisters or calluses. Without treatment and/or prevention it will worsen to become broken skin with the inner layers of the skin becoming damaged. Eventually the skin breakdown becomes an open sore or wound and is classified as a foot ulcer. At this stage there could be damage to muscle, tendons and even bones. Infection of the foot ulcer makes the heath problem much worse.

A DEVELOPING FOOT ULCER

HOT SPOT   **BROKEN SKIN**

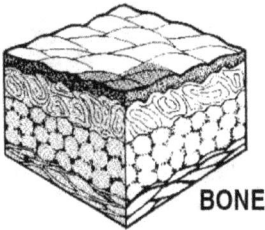 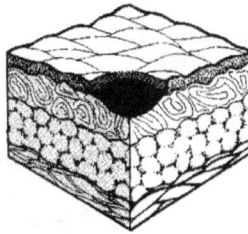

BONE

GETTING WORSE   **SERIOUS ULCER**

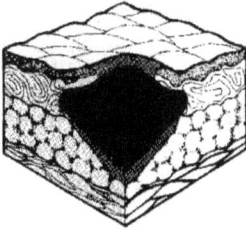 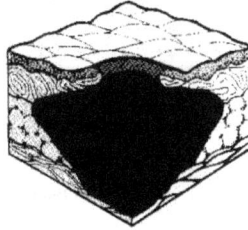

SOMETHING TO THINK ABOUT...

A foot ulcer can be likened to an
iceberg where most of the damage
lies below the surface of the skin.

THE DANGER SIGNS

DIABETIC FOOT ULCER QUIZ

Symptom/Observation: Check if experienced

R   L

❑   ❑ Loss of feeling in your foot when you touch it

❑   ❑ An open sore or wound that doesn't heal within 7 days

❑   ❑ Anything unusual on your foot such as:

        ❑ blister ❑ crack ❑ callus ❑ corn

        ❑ discolored toenails

❑   ❑ Burning sensation or a foot that feels too warm and dry

❑   ❑ Changes in shape, e.g. cocked-up toe

❑   ❑ Socks or hosiery that has blood or fluid stains

❑   ❑ Signs of infection such as: ❑ swelling ❑ pain

        ❑ redness ❑ fever ❑ fluid

        ❑ drainage ❑ odor

The previous pages have been a brief introduction to the problem of foot ulcers. Before we go any further with regard to treatment and prevention it will be useful to look at the foot more thoroughly as a vital, although somewhat unappreciated, part of the body.

You hardly ever think of your feet when they are working well. In our culture the foot is one of the least glamorous parts of the body. Having said that there are other cultures where the feet are revered and ritually cared for. In the western world, however, even your average dyed-in-the-wool hypochondriac will avoid complaining about feet; he or she will choose much more imaginative symptoms like headaches, stomach problems or palpitations of the heart. Nobody wants to be known as having problems with their feet.

And yet, how many times have you heard someone say, "My feet are killing me"? The truth is that most of us only appreciate our feet when something goes wrong with them – at that point they become the most important part of our bodies!

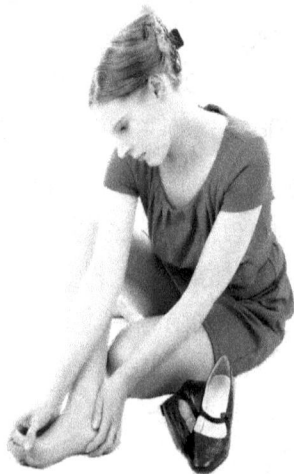

DID YOU KNOW...

The average person in his or her
lifetime will walk 120,000 miles,
or almost 5 times around the
circumference of the earth!

ANATOMY OF THE FOOT

The foot contains 26 bones six principal ligaments, bands of fibrous tissue, numerous muscles and a complicated system of arteries and veins, all of which is, of course, surrounded by skin. The various bones serve many functions including locomotion, balance, protection and weight bearing.

This sophisticated and complex system is designed in such a way as to form a longitudinal arch, which absorbs the shock of walking, together with a transverse arch which helps to distribute weight. The heel bone helps support this longitudinal foot arch.

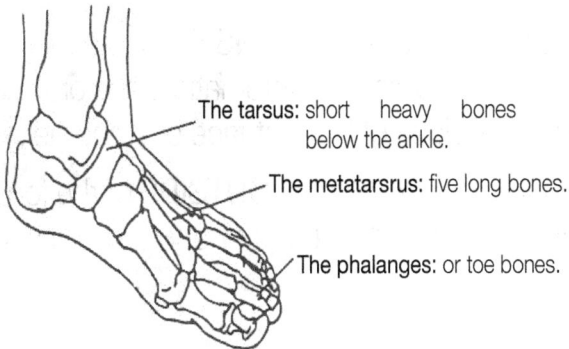

The tarsus: short heavy bones below the ankle.

The metatarsrus: five long bones.

The phalanges: or toe bones.

Below are some simple drawings which indicate common names used by the health care team when referring to the foot.

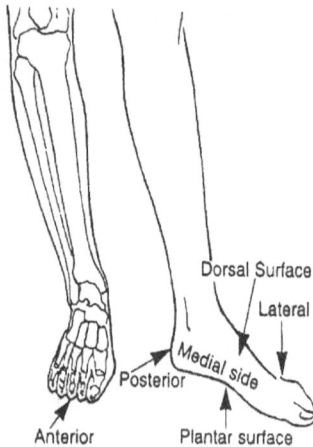

Now let's appreciate the significance of these drawings.

The **dorsal** view is the **TOP** of the foot. Obviously the toenails are usually seen on the dorsal view of the foot.

The **plantar** view of the foot is the **BOTTOM** of the foot. Plantar ulcers or warts are found at the bottom of the foot. This is also the most common area for foot ulcers.

The **medial** view is on the **INSIDE** of the foot. This is where you may find symptomatic discoloration. The two medial sides of the feet face one another.

The **lateral** view is on the **OUTSIDE** of the foot. This is the thinnest part of the foot and faces away from the body.

Anterior view describes a location in front and forward. A good example would be your face or tummy.

Posterior view describes a location toward the rear or behind. Your back or bottom would be an example.

Other important words to know are:

Proximal: this means "near to" a part of your body. For example, your ankle is more proximal to your leg than your big toe.

Distal: this means "farther from" a part of your body. Using the same example, you would say your big toe is more distal to your leg than your ankle.

Superficial: this means nearer the surface. If a pressure ulcer isn't superficial it's deep, as in a scratch that is either superficial or deep (heavily bleeding).

So when a physician or nurse says you have a superficial plantar ulcer proximate to the big toe, it means you have an ulcer which is not deep, is close to the surface of the skin and is located at the bottom of the foot near to the big toe.

INTRODUCING DIABETES

Diabetes is a chronic disorder that causes high blood sugar (hyperglycemia).

Sugar (glucose) is the fuel that gives cells energy. The body produces a hormone called insulin that assists the cells in the body to use the sugar. It is this insulin which helps the glucose level in the blood keep within normal levels.

High blood sugar develops when the body is unable to produce or use insulin properly and this is the essence of the diabetes condition.

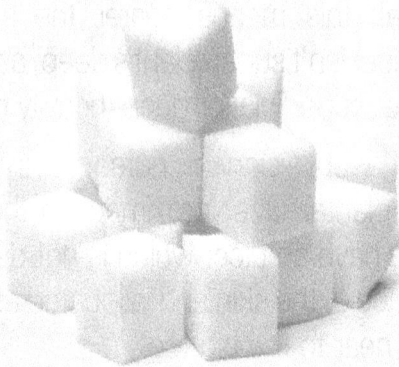

This defensive reaction on the part of the body to get its blood sugar or glucose levels back to normal can create one or more of the following symptoms.

SYMPTOMS OF DIABETES

❑ EXCESSIVE THIRST

❑ FATIGUE, WEAKNESS

❑ WEIGHT LOSS

❑ INCREASED APPETITE

❑ INFECTIONS

❑ SLOW HEALING OF WOUNDS

❑ ITCHING

❑ CHANGES IN VISION

❑ NUMBNESS, PAIN OR TINGLING IN THE HANDS OR FEET

There are almost 30 million people in North America with diabetes and there are many millions of people that have diabetes who do not know they have the disease.

Again, the common denominator among people with diabetes is high blood sugar. The good news is that they can use a monitor on a daily basis to check the level of blood sugar and thereby control their sugar levels through treatment and life style choices.

GLUCOSE MONITORING

A glucose monitor is used to test blood sugar levels. The tip of the finger is pricked for a drop of blood. The blood is then applied to a test strip and the monitor reads the strip.

Keeping blood glucose readings within the normal levels helps prevent a foot ulcer developing or getting worse.

The recommended blood glucose values differ depending on the time that the person ate. For example, the desired range will be lower before eating and higher within two hours of eating a meal.

Physicians will advise patients on preferred individual blood glucose levels but the normal healthy levels after a meal are 5–10 mmol/L. In the UK, using a different measurement system, the levels are 60-115 mg/dL

These glucose blood level numbers appear on the monitor and this aid becomes a very important part of everyday management of diabetes because you can make changes in diet, lifestyle or medication to adjust these glucose levels.

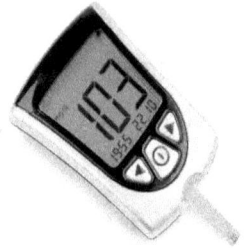

You may be taught how to do glucose monitoring at home or in a health care facility. If you are a health

worker you may be required to do the test if your client is unable to do it. You may also be required to keep good records of the times and results of the tests, although many glucose meters now have the technology to display past readings.

In any event, you should be aware of this procedure and encourage your clients to carry out the practice. As keeping blood glucose levels normal is very important to preventing and even healing a diabetic foot ulcer, you should try to champion this practice, seeking feedback from clients and praising them for their efforts.

HOW DIABETES CONTRIBUTES
TO A FOOT ULCER

You now know that the effect of diabetes is to increase the levels of blood sugar (glucose). This increased blood sugar level contributes in the following two ways to the development of foot ulcers:

NERVE DAMAGE: Known medically as peripheral neuropathy (PN for short), this is a breakdown or disorder of your nerves near the surface of your feet. ("Peripheral" means near the surface and "neuropathy" means disorder of the nerves.) The exact incidence of PN is difficult to assess. However it is estimated that 10% to 20% of people with diabetes have PN; as the years pass, this figure can increase to over 50%.

BLOOD CIRCULATION PROBLEMS: Known medically as peripheral arterial disease (PAD for short), this simply means problems with the blood circulation system near the surface of your feet. Another word your medical team may use for this problem is ischemia, which means poor blood supply. Keeping in mind that "peripheral" means near the surface while arterial relates to the arteries, you can see that PAD is a disease near the surface, related to the arteries. Sometimes the medical team may say peripheral vascular disease, and in this case "vascular" means all blood vessels (including veins) instead of just arterial.

These two factors are the primary reasons for foot ulcers associated with diabetes. One of these problems may dominate but the cause of a foot ulcer is always a combination of both nerve damage and blood circulatory problems. By understanding how these two conditions – PN and PAD – contribute to foot ulcers, you will have a greater understanding of the treatment and be knowledgeable on preventing and treating the problem.

THE INSENSITIVE FOOT

The bottom line of both these conditions (PN and PAD) is that they can make the foot insensitive. This means that normal sensations like pain, heat, cold, trauma, irritations or even just a light touch are sometimes difficult to feel. This insensitivity can lead to damage to the foot which in turn can create the development of a foot ulcer.

Pain is nature's way of warning that something is wrong and must be attended to. Under normal circumstances, for instance, a person with a small stone lodged in her shoe will soon feel the protuberance and sense the irritation being caused, take off the shoe and remove the stone. However an insensitive (sometimes called insensate) foot may not feel the pain and serious damage may be done to the skin over time because the stone remains and continues to irritate the skin.

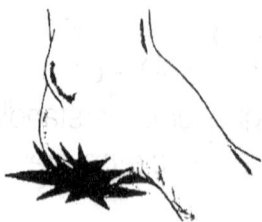

PARTS OF THE FOOT AT RISK

From the previous explanations you would expect the pressure points of the foot would be the most vulnerable. The diagram shows where foot ulcers can develop most easily.

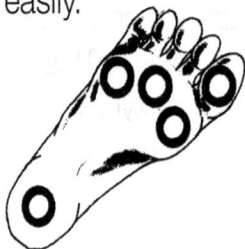

OTHER RISK FACTORS

We should now appreciate that the high blood sugar caused by diabetes is the greatest causative factor in developing an insensitive foot prone or at risk to developing a foot ulcer. This is the number one risk factor.

There are other risk factors, some medical such as high blood pressure, high cholesterol levels, blood circulation disorders and not having regular screening for diabetes. These are all the responsibility of the medical team.

It is worth noting that early diagnosis of diabetes is vital; there are so many people who have diabetes without knowing it because in the early stages there are few obvious symptoms. The quicker you are diagnosed the less chance of diabetic complications such as foot problems occurring.

Some risk factors such as heredity (the predisposition of a person to have diabetes) and old age are uncontrollable – there's nothing you can do about them. However, there are some risk factors you can help minimize, by good foot care practices such as:

• Making sure regular foot inspection takes place

• Quitting smoking

• Physical exercise

- Good nutrition to help weight loss
- Maintaining optimum hygiene to avoid foot infection
- Adherence to treatment
- Ensuring early diagnosis of diabetes by having regular check-ups

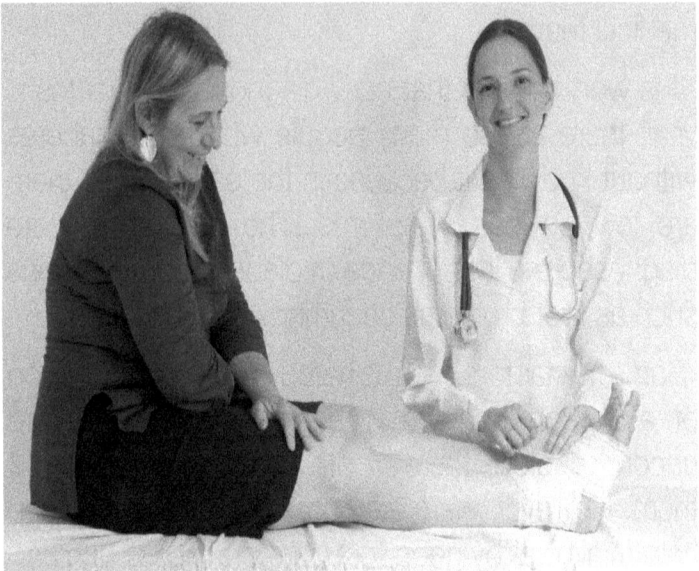

FOOT CARE PRACTICES

Remember that most serious foot problems start with injury or excessive pressure on the blood vessels. Good foot care practices, however, can help mitigate the damage and prevent a serious foot ulcer from developing.

You may be involved directly with foot care or you may simply have an appreciation of foot care principles. Either way, you can help prevent a foot ulcer developing or help in the healing process there is an existing foot ulcer.

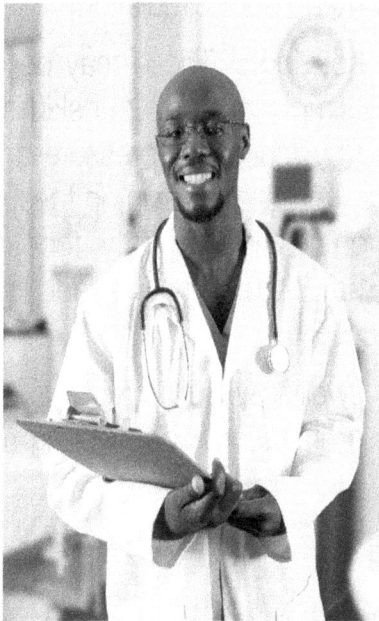

INSPECTION

- Check daily for blisters, cuts, scratches or sores, all potential problems that your physician or nurse must know about.

- Check for dryness and cracks. This is a sign the skin is breaking down, which can allow bacteria or fungi to grow, increasing the risk of infection.

- Check for corns and calluses. These have to be treated by a professional. Never try to treat or remove them yourself!

- Check for any changes in color. Redness with streaks is often a sign of infection. Pale or blue tones may mean poor circulation.

- Check for hot spots. These may be colored red or you may simply feel that your skin is hot. These are caused by friction or pressure and can turn into blisters, corns (thick skin on toes), or calluses (thick skin on the bottom of the foot). Conversely, cold feet may be a sign the feet aren't getting enough blood.

- Check for swelling which may be a sign of poor circulation or infection. The swelling may also be tender.

- If necessary, use a mirror to see the bottom of the feet.

- Check between the toes for fungal infection, cracks and other problems.

- Inspect feet in good lighting.

- Inspect the insides of shoes for foreign objects, nail points, torn lining, cracks and rough areas. Make sure foot powder has not accumulated and caked because this can be a source of irritation.

- If someone has impaired vision make sure the foot is checked by a health worker or family member.

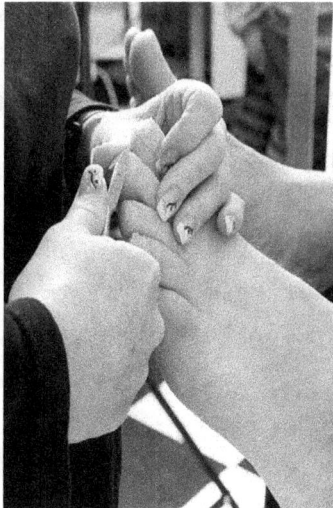

DAILY WASH AND DRY

- Feet should be washed every day to help avoid infection.

- Feet should not be soaked for long periods of time. This will make them vulnerable, depleting them of their protective natural oils.

- Always use a mild soap. Heavily perfumed soap can cause irritation or allergic reactions.

- Use warm water, not hot. Hot water can traumatize the feet making them vulnerable to infection. Test the water with your hand before immersing the feet.

- Dry well, but no hard rubbing or using a rough towel. Make sure the area between the toes is dried well but do make sure the towel is not used aggressively.

- You can use a little powder for sweaty/perspiring feet. You may use non perfumed powder, talcum powder or cornstarch to help keep feet dry. Do not let powder cake, especially between the toes.

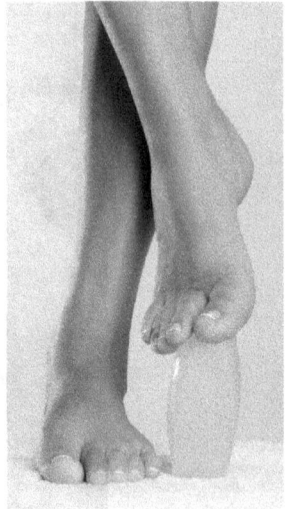

SKIN CARE AND LUBRICATION

- Get advice from the nurse or physician or abide by the facility policies about which lubricating lotion, oil or cream to use.

- Do not put lotion in open sores or between the toes.

- Avoid perfumed lotions because of the potential problems of irritation and allergic reactions.

- Apply the lotion only after bathing and drying the feet. This will help maintain moisture and help with dry skin.

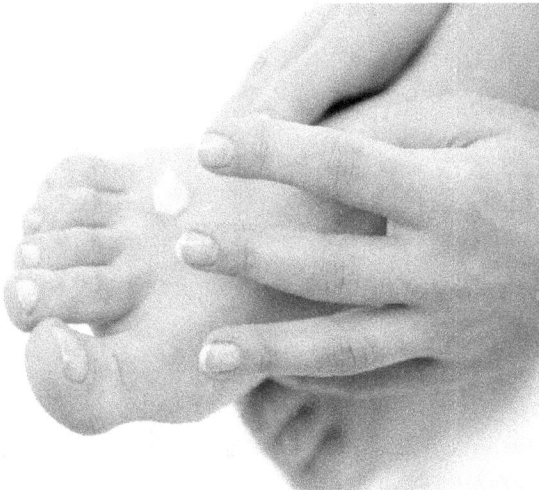

TOENAIL CARE

- Cutting toenails should be done with clean nail clippers, not scissors.

- Toenails are softer after bathing and easier to cut.

- Cut straight across. Do not cut the nail shorter than the fleshy part and do not curve the sides of the nail.

- Make sure the lighting is bright.

- Do not explore corners of the toe with sharp instruments.

- Avoid cuts as these could cause infections.

- If the nails tend to grow in, a very small piece of cotton inserted into the corners can sometimes help.

- If the toenails are thick, curved or extremely hard, do not take a chance. Inform the health care professional.

- If tissue around the nail is injured, the application of a cotton swab can cleanse this area.

- Cleansing with a soft brush will remove accumulations of unwanted tissue in the nail groove.

- Remove sharp edges only with a nail file or emery board.

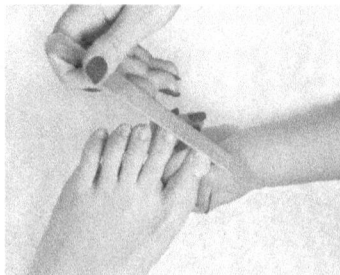

SHOES AND SOCKS

- Purchase shoes that are comfortable at the time of purchase. Do not depend on them to stretch after wearing them for a while.

- Shoes should be made of leather.

- Purchase shoes late in the afternoon when your feet are at their largest. They should feel comfortable at the time of purchase.

- Purchase shoes that offer good protection – hard soles and soft tops. Women should avoid high heels and pointed toes.

- Purchase shoes from a medical specialist shop or a store that understands your needs.

- Wear new shoes for a couple of hours at a time during the first five days to give them a chance to break in properly.

- Never buy shoes with build-ups or corrective pads without the advice of your health care professional.

- Ideally, try to change your shoes during the day. That way you are never in one pair long enough to cause any serious damage.

- Any running or special walking shoes should be purchased only after liaison with your physician or orthotist.

- Socks must be seamless, they must never have been mended and they must be properly fitted. If you get a hole in your sock, throw it out.

- Do not purchase socks or panty hose that are tight. They could affect your blood circulation.

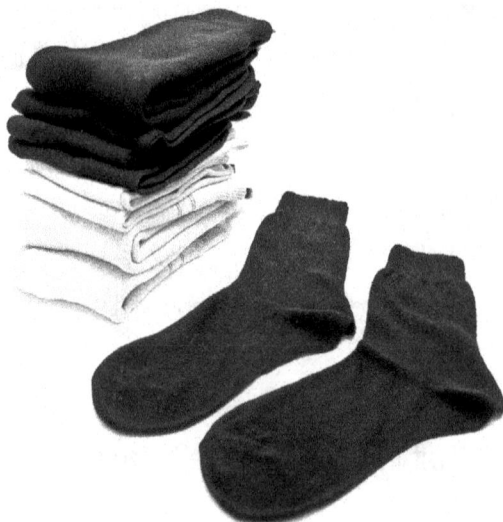

- Chose clean cotton socks. Cotton allows your feet to "breathe" and prevents sweating.

- Change socks daily. If washing socks by hand, make sure all the soap has been rinsed out of the sock.

- Never wear two pairs of socks to keep warm. Creases can occur and cause skin damage.

WALKING TIPS

Unless advised otherwise by the doctor, walking is generally good for the feet. It improves circulation and psychologically it is important to maintain independence, no matter what your age.

Here are some tips:

- Always walk with shoe wear, never barefoot. The surface of the skin must be protected at all times.

- Avoid walking on hot surfaces like sandy beaches or the cement around a swimming pool.

- Always wear socks with your shoes for the skin protection they provide. A slight protrusion in a shoe can be more devastating without socks.

- Never wear sandals with thongs between the toes. They can traumatize your skin.

- In winter always wear warm footwear, with cotton socks or fleece-lined boots.

- Walk on level ground.

- Use slippers when you get out of bed.

- Make sure lights are on in dark rooms, hallways and stairways.

- Take extra care on icy streets and sidewalks.

- Use your cane or walker, if necessary, or walk with a friend or family member.

- If it's hot, stay in a shaded area and try to avoid the sun. You may misjudge how hot it really is.

- Do not walk when you have pain or open sores that rub on clothes or shoes.

- If your legs and feet hurt after walking, stop and rest for a while.

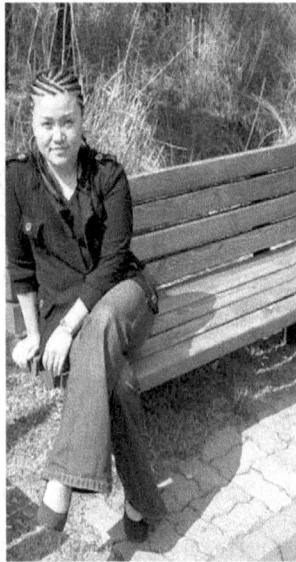

PITFALLS TO FOOT CARE

The following are some of the most common mistakes people make, causing problems with their feet:

- Do not cut corns or calluses or use chemical agents, corn plasters or strong antiseptic solutions them. Any of these can put the feet at risk of infection. Always see a health care professional for this sort of care.

- Do not use heating pads, electric blankets or hot water bottles on your feet at night in bed. This can overheat the feet, cause sweating and increase the risk of damage and infection. Alternately, use socks at night to keep warm.

- Do not wear sandals or flip-flops. These can cause trauma and injury in between the toes and there is a potential for slipping. Always wear sensible casual shoes with proper protective qualities.

FOOT ULCER TREATMENT

The core to all of the treatment options is glucose control or lowering your blood sugars to a normal range through insulin, medication, diet and exercise.

However the following actions are needed in treating diabetic foot problems:

WOUND CARE

This is the domain of the nurse, physician or other health care professional. They will assess the ulcer and choose the appropriate dressing and other treatments to ensure healing. Here are some of the activities the health care professional will carry out to achieve healing:

Assessment

Your clinician must first assess and document the wound as to its size, how much exudates (drainage) is occurring, the type of tissue present, the level of pain the wound is causing and the condition of the skin at the wound edge.

Blood flow

This is an extremely important factor that will help the clinician assess the probability of healing and/or the length of time it may take to heal the foot ulcer.

If the ulcer is going to heal, it has to have supplies of nutrients from blood around the infected area. Poor blood flow or circulation will make matters more difficult.

Some of the symptoms of poor blood circulation include:

- Pain or cramping of the calves
- Pain in the legs at night or at rest
- Loss of leg hair and thickened toe nails
- Cold feet with loss of pulses

Debridement

Debridement often means removing dead tissue like scabs which can slow down the healing process. It is done to make sure the wound tissue is in the best possible condition to heal.

Dressing selection (to maintain moisture balance)

The objectives of a dressing are to provide the correct balance of moisture for diabetic foot ulcers and also minimize trauma and risk of infection. Your clinician is trained to have a good understanding of the various dressing categories and their characteristics in order to match the dressing needs of the person with the diabetic foot ulcer.

The best analogy for the right moisture of a wound is to liken the wound to the moisture levels on the surface of the eye.

Here are some of the guidelines used in making the right decision on dressing choices:

- Objective and comprehensive assessment including exudate level, bacterial balance and need for debridement.

- Consider a dressing or combination of dressings that matches the needs of the wound assessment.

- Attempt to keep the wound bed continuously moist and the edge of the wound dry.

- Avoid drying out the wound – simply control the exudates.

- Avoid wound "dead space" by filling cavities with dressing material.

- Consideration of the caregiver's time.

- An improving diabetic foot ulcer wound usually has a pink wound bed and an advancing (shrinking) wound margin.

INFECTION CONTROL

When it comes to foot care it is essential to make sure the worst eventuality does not occur – an infection within the ulcer.

People with diabetes are hospitalized for foot infections more often than for any other complication; such infections are the cause of most of the foot amputations that take place.

Therefore, it's worth taking the time to understand how an infection can start and what must be done to stop it progressing.

Diabetic foot ulcers have bacteria "colonized" within the ulcer. Usually the healing process and body fluids can stabilize and deal with the microbes/bacteria without causing any problem in the healing process. However, if the bacteria count becomes disproportionate, the wound may show signs of distress and healing will be impaired.

Often debridement (removing dead tissue) can solve the problem by removing the environment for bacteria/microbe growth. If debridement is insufficient to control the critical colonization of the wound surface, then topical antimicrobials may be used for a maximum of two weeks.

Failure to improve the wound environment at this time would indicate the need for wide spectrum oral antibiotics to eradicate all possible problem bacteria/microbes to ensure no survival advantage is given to a specific bacteria/microbe strain.

Effective foot inspection, disciplined foot care and making sure of compliance to treatment (e.g. taking antibiotics) are the three activities you can do to prevent an infection occurring.

If you allow the skin on the feet to become compromised or vulnerable, bacteria can find an easy access to the debilitated skin and launch a destructive campaign against the foot.

PRESSURE DOWNLOADING

When a foot has lost its protective (feeling) sensations the health care professional will sometimes prescribe a "pressure downloading" device which will remove any destructive pressure of the foot.

Some people may use a removable walker as shown here or they may have a "total contact cast" which is a customized cast (just like with a fracture) to absolutely prevent any pressure on the foot.

In some cases, a person may have special shoes or sandals to achieve this benefit.

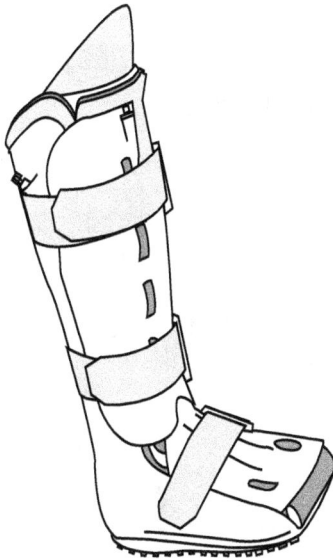

EDUCATION

There are three types of patients who can benefit from health education and preventative actions. They are as follows:

1. Diabetic patient who is fit and healthy and whose feet are not at risk.

- Regular foot inspection
- Good foot hygiene
- Prompt treatment of athlete's foot or other fungal infections
- Careful care and maintenance of the toenails

2. Diabetic patient whose feet are at risk but is otherwise fit and active.

- All of the points in the checklist above.
- Foot assessment for pressure points & vigilance on these areas.
- Regular chiropody/podiatrist nail care and debridement of calluses.
- Advice on avoiding traumatic injury, e.g. hot bathwater, cuts, grazes, etc.

3. Diabetic patient who is frail, whose feet are at risk, and who is dependant on others.

- All of the above but with the help of a caregiver.

- Complete orthotic/chiropody and/or podiatry services.

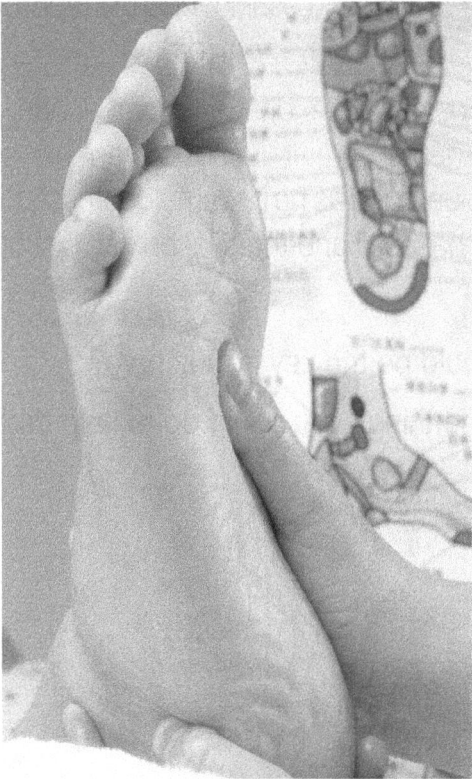

CASE EXAMPLE

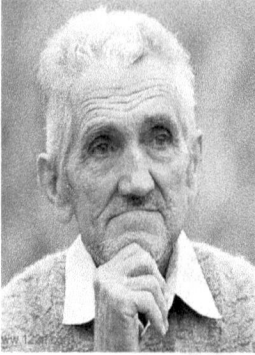

Mr. Simpson is an 82-year-old, well-educated gentleman who has had diabetes for 26 years and now lives in a long term care facility. One month ago he developed a diabetic foot ulcer on his big toe which requires a dressing change approximately every third day.

Mr. Simpson's wife died 6 months ago and he became depressed; it is suspected his self care practices declined as he became depressed. He likes to watch baseball and the season has just started.

What could be the key issues here?

List some things you could do to help this client.

YOUR ANSWERS TO CASE EXAMPLE

SUGGESTED ANSWERS TO CASE EXAMPLE

Because Mr. Simpson's self care practices have declined since his wife died, his depression may have caused him not to practice foot care. As well, his glucose control may now be poor, his nutrition may have faltered and he may not be exercising as much. He may be at risk for more ulcers developing or a deterioration of the existing ulcer. Overall motivation and morale could be the common denominator.

You could do some of the following:

a) Inspect his feet to look for signs of other ulcers.

b) Demonstrate what he has to do to maintain good foot care

c) As he is well educated, explain the quality of life benefits of looking after yourself.

d) Ask about his glucose monitoring (appeal to his achievement motives of maintaining control).

e) Offer a reward, e.g., plenty of baseball games to watch if you can "get about" better.

CONCLUSION

Prevention is the key to foot health; if you are a front line health worker dealing with at risk people with diabetes, you are best positioned to apply a human, influential touch to helping the person deal with all the issues.

Try not to be overwhelmed by all the variables – you can only do so much. Foot care, inspection of the foot, encouraging glucose control when appropriate, presenting positive lifestyle issues (like not smoking), and ensuring good hygiene are some of the important contributions you can make within the framework of your job.

If you work for a facility, management absolutely depends on you to ensure quality care for the client. In the developing age of facility inspections and objective quality standards being formulated and assessed, your role is vital for the well being of your organization.

If you are a person with a foot ulcer or are at risk of developing one, just understanding this health issue, its causes and the common sense ways of maintaining healthy feet can make a dramatic impact on your foot health.

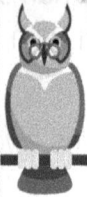

CHECK YOUR KNOWLEDGE

1. What is the major characteristic of diabetes?

2. What is the complication of diabetes that can lead to an amputation?

3. Name two useful foot care practices?

4. Why is an infection of the foot to be avoided at all costs?

5. How many times a week should a foot be inspected for someone with diabetes at risk for a foot ulcer?

TEST YOURSELF

Please circle to indicate the best answer:

1. What answer does NOT apply to diabetes?

a. It can cause many different complications such as eye, kidney, cardiovascular and skin problems.

b. It is characterized by high blood sugars.

c. Lifestyle issues such as being overweight can contribute to causing diabetes.

d. As soon as diabetes develops in a person, the symptoms are dramatic and obvious.

2. Which of the following causes do NOT contribute to developing a foot ulcer?

a. A numb or insensitive foot

b. Poor blood circulation

c. Nerve damage

d. Constantly standing up in a job

3. Which treatment is NOT appropriate for healing a diabetic foot ulcer?

a. Wound dressings

b. Quitting smoking

c. Blood sugar control

d. Blood thinning medication

4. What aspect of healing the foot ulcer do you consider most important in the short term?

a. Overall foot care

b. Glucose control

c. Cholesterol control

d. Losing weight

5. Why is infection important to avoid in a foot ulcer?

a. The cost of antibiotics can be very expensive.

b. It can slow healing or lead to amputation.

c. It will require more visits from the health care professional.

d. Other clients can become infected.

6. What should be done if someone complains of feet being cold during sleep?

a. Use a heating pad

b. Use a hot water bottle

c. Put on a pair of socks

d. Use an electric blanket

7. What should be done if a foot has a corn or callus?

a. Purchase and apply a chemical agent from a pharmacy.

b. Gently use scissors to remove provided there is little or no pain.

c. See a health professional for treatment.

d. Use a well proven antiseptic.

ANSWERS

1. d. People can have diabetes for many years without any obvious symptoms.

2. d. Constantly standing up in a job may contribute to varicose veins but the other three points mentioned can contribute to a diabetic foot ulcer.

3. d. There is no evidence that blood thinning medication helps but all the other three are important treatment factors.

4. a. Overall foot care can provide the healing environment and prevent dangerous infections. The other three answers are correct but for the long term.

5. b. Infection can slow healing or lead to amputation; these are serious implications of infection that outweigh anything else.

6. c. Socks are the most sensible alternative – the others can cause complications through sweating, damage or infection.

7. c. Always see a health professional; doing any of the other things listed can cause complications.

Foot Care Bibliography

Ahroni JH. Teaching foot care creatively and successfully. Diabetes Ed.1993; 19:320-S

American Diabetes Association. Standards of Medical care in Diabetes-2007. Diabetes Care. 2007; 30 (Suppl.): S4-S41

Boulton A. The Diabetic Foot Epidemiology, Risk Factors and the Status of Care. Diabetes Voice.2005;50 (special issue)

Bus SA, Valk GD, van Deursen RW et al. The effectiveness of footwear and offloading interventions to prevent and heal foot ulcers.. Diabetes Metb. Res Rev.2008;24 (suppl.)S162-S180

Canadian Diabetes Association. Clinical Practice Guidelines for the Management of Diabetes. Canadian J Diabetes 2008u;31 (suppl.1) S1-S201.

Eneroth M, Larson J, Oscarsson c, Nutritional Supplementation for diabetic Foot Ulcers: the first RCT. Wound Care 2004;13 (6):230-234

Inlow S. Sixty second foot exam for people with diabetes. Wound Care Canada 2004; 2 (2): 10-11

Lorimer D, French et al. Neale's Disorders of the Foot, seventh edition New York: Churchill Livingstone.2006

National Institute for Health and Clinical Excellence. Type 2 Diabetes. Prevention and Management of Foot Problems. Clinical Guideline 10. London, UK: National Institute for Clinical Excellence.

Registered Nurses Association of Ontario (RNAO) Nursing Best Practice Guideline: reducing foot complications of people with diabetes.-revised 2007. Toronto ON.

Singh N, Armstrong DG,:Lipsky BA. Preventing foot ulcers in patients with Diabetes. JAMA. 2005;293 (2): 217-218

Valk GD, kriegsman DM, Assendelft WJ Patient education for preventing diabetic foot ulceration. Cochrane database System Review 2005; 5:CD001488

www.ingramcontent.com/pod-product-compliance
Lightning Source LLC
Chambersburg PA
CBHW060640280326
41933CB00012B/2098